Celebrate the Win!

Celebrate the Win!

STEMI, Widow Maker, and the Miracle After

Henry Cross

(To be used alongside Taylor's Gift and 31 Days of Grace)

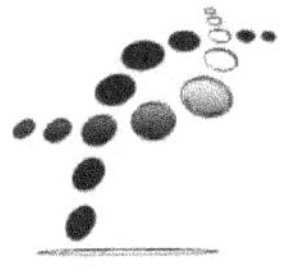

AeA Publishing

Visit the author's website online at henrycross.org

Visit Taylor's Gift Farm at TaylorsGiftFarm.org

AeA Publishing, the AeA logo, and *Taylor's Gift* are trademarks of Advisory Engineering & Analytics, LLC.

AeA Publishing is the non-fiction imprint of Advisory Engineering & Analytics, LLC., Frisco, Texas.

Taylor's Gift: Living Life Perfectly in the Present

Designed and Edited by Henry Cross.

Edited using ChatGPT, Grammarly, and Antigravity artificial intelligence tools as enhancements to ensure consistency, correct grammar, and tone of voice presented.

Songs written and edited using ChatGPT and Suno.com. Henry does not sing or play instruments, but he has used these tools to bring his words to life through music.

For information about special discounts for bulk purchases, please contact AeA Publishing at publisher@henrycross.org.

ISBN 979-8-9957207-2-0 (Hardback)

ISBN 979-8-9957207-4-4 (paperback)

"The text of this manuscript was authored by Henry. Artificial intelligence tools, including ChatGPT, Grammarly, and Antigravity, were utilized specifically for editing and enhancement purposes—ensuring consistency, correcting grammar, and refining the tone of voice."

"Companion songs were written with lyrics by Henry, while the music and vocals were composed and produced using ChatGPT and Suno.com. Henry does not sing or play instruments and utilized these tools to bring his written words to life through music."

Contents

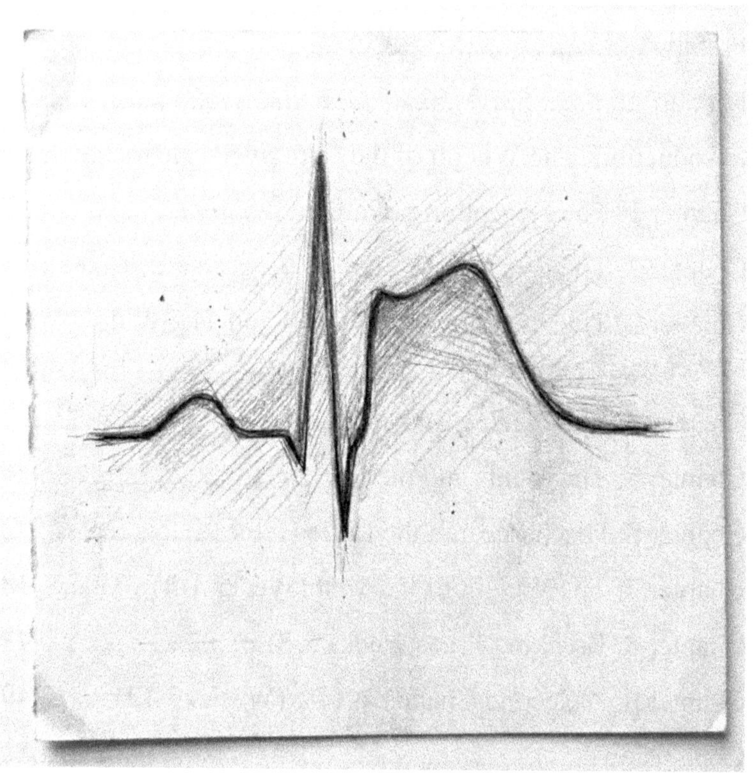

Prelude

I have written this supplemental short story as a companion to *Taylor's Gift*, focusing on a profound truth often left unspoken: true caregivers instinctively bury their own needs beneath the survival and comfort of those they love. We sacrifice sleep, health, and peace of mind without a second thought. Yet, the reality is that no one is invincible. While not every caregiver will suffer a heart attack in the dead of night, every single one of us will eventually face a sudden, unavoidable crisis that shatters our ability to simply 'carry on.' *Taylor's Gift* is dedicated to these selfless souls—the caregivers who know the profound physical and emotional risks of their calling, yet courageously press into the darkness, day after demanding day."

Forward

There is a quiet, unspoken weight that every caregiver carries. It is an abstract, terrifying question that lingers in the back of the mind during the quiet moments of the day, creeping into our thoughts just as we drift off to sleep: *What happens when the caregiver needs care?*

This is a fear I know intimately. Since my divorce, I have been a single parent and the sole caregiver for my daughter, Taylor. Our dynamic is built on a foundation of profound love, unwavering routine, and absolute presence. My daily life is structured to ensure that Taylor's world remains safe, vibrant, and fully supported.

But beneath that structured life at our quiet East Texas farmhouse, the silent worry has always hummed in the background. What if a sudden crisis physically prevents me from being present? What if something strikes without warning, ripping me away from the very person I am entirely responsible for protecting? What happens when the caregiver needs care?

This book is directly written for those of you who know exactly what that fear feels like. It is for the caregivers, the single parents, the spouses, and the protectors who lie awake at night calculating contingencies, organizing legal documents, and silently praying that they are never suddenly incapacitated. You meticulously label "Go-Kits" and build detailed notebooks just in case someone else ever needs to step into your shoes. You do everything humanly possible to plan for the unthinkable.

I was exactly like you. I had the plans. I had the duplicates. I had the sheer force of will to push through stress and exhaustion to ensure Taylor's life never skipped a beat.

Then, the unthinkable arrived.

On the night of December 16, 2025, the abstract fear I had lived with for years transformed into a terrifying, physical reality. A massive, catastrophic heart attack—a Widow Maker—struck me in the dead of the night inside our isolated farmhouse, while Taylor slept peacefully just down the hall.

This story is an honest, unvarnished account of what happens when the caregiver is abruptly forced to fight for their own survival. It is a journey through severe physical trauma, the agonizing conflict between self-preservation and caregiving duties, and the miraculous, humbling road to recovery. But above all, it is a testament to the fact that while we cannot predict the crisis, we can rely on an abundance of grace when the darkest moment finally arrives.

Introduction: The Weight of the Caregiver's Heart

There is a profound stillness that descends upon a Texas farmhouse in the dead of night in December. It isn't just an absence of sound; it is a heavy, almost tangible silence that settles over the pastures, freezing the dew on the grass and turning the night air into something sharp and brittle. On the evening of December 16, 2025, that stillness held the farmhouse in a deep embrace. Inside, however, the warmth of the home was defined by something much stronger than the heater humming in the corner. It was defined by Taylor.

If you have read *Taylor's Gift*, you know that my life is inextricably bound to hers. To perfectly describe Taylor to someone who hasn't met her is like trying to describe the precise color of a sunset; words often fall short. When she walks into a room—or into places like Aspire Day Habilitation in Lewisville, Texas—she is greeted with the kind of joy and familiarity that television sets aside for its favorite characters. They shout her name like everyone's favorite regular at *Cheers*. She has a capacity for love and an intuition that often defies typical clinical assessments. She bounces through life, full of innocence, lighting up the corners of my world.

Yet, being her caregiver carries a silent, immutable weight. It is a responsibility that quietly rewires a person's priorities, shifting the center of gravity away from one's own self and squarely onto the shoulders of another. Every decision, from the mundane to the monumental, is filtered through a single, defining question: *How will this affect Taylor?*

When you love someone who depends on you entirely, you develop a subtle, chronic fear. It isn't a loud, paralyzing terror, but a quiet whisper that lingers at the back of your mind, especially in the quiet hours of a cold winter night. *What happens to her if something happens to me?*

You push that thought down. You build routines. You lean into the strength of your community—your family, your neighbors, your friends. You rely on people like Chris, who watches the farm and the animals, or Richard, Luis, Chuck, and Fred. You take comfort in the network of love that surrounds you. But at the end of the day, when the lights go out and the darkness settles over the pasture, you are the final line of defense. You are the caregiver. You are the anchor.

I didn't know it yet, but that night, my anchor was about to break.

The year had brought its typical share of challenges and triumphs. We were looking forward to the simple joys of the upcoming Christmas season. I was a man who planned his days meticulously. OCD, some might jokingly call it, but the precision was necessary. There is no room for error when another human being relies on your consistency. I worried about the stock market, I stressed over the news, and I meticulously maintained the farmhouse, always ensuring the water in the tank out in the pasture was completely free of ice for Suny and the livestock.

The illusion of control is a powerful sedative. We convince ourselves that if we eat right, act responsibly, and check all the boxes on our daily to-do lists, we are immune to the sudden, violent interruptions of fate. We believe our bodies will politely inform us if something is slowly shifting out of alignment.

But life, and the mortal vessels we inhabit, rarely adhere to our schedules.

There are moments in life that act as hard dividers. A definitive *Before* and an unalterable *After*. December 16, 2025, was my threshold. It was the night that forced me to confront the absolute fragility of my own existence, the chaotic reality of a failing body, and the miraculous, enduring grace of a God who knew me long before I ever needed to call out His name in desperation.

This book is the chronicling of that *After*. It is the story of a Widow Maker, a 1500-pound mule that tried to kick the life out of my chest, a defective wearable defibrillator I affectionately and frustratingly came to call my "little helper," and the first one hundred days of a second chance at life. But mostly, it is a story about the stubborn, unyielding priority of love, and the realization that sometimes the caregiver must learn how to be the one who is cared for.

Chapter 1: The Deception of Pain

The clock reads 9:15 PM.

The farmhouse felt normal, insulated against the dropping temperatures for the night in East Texas. Taylor had settled into the evening's rhythm, the quiet comfort of our home providing a familiar backdrop. Everything was routine, predictable, safe. We drove to Dallas earlier this day and arrived home just around 8:00 pm. Taylor went to bed, and I sat down to read the mail and catch a few minutes of the evening news. Shortly thereafter, I went to bed too.

Then, the first sensation arrived.

It wasn't the cinematic clutch of the chest, nor the dramatic collapse that television dramas condition us to expect. It was insidious. It began as a vague, hollow ache—a slow, simmering discomfort resting stubbornly in my upper abdomen.

Food poisoning, my mind immediately deduced. Or perhaps severe indigestion.

It is fascinating how the human brain will grasp at the most mundane explanation to avoid confronting a terrifying reality. Denial is the first, desperate defense mechanism of a body falling into crisis. I mentally retraced my day, searching for the culprit. A bad piece of meat at lunch or that drive-through order in Mt. Pleasant on the way home? Something I drank from the cup that had been in the truck all day long? The discomfort was irritating, distracting me from the quiet peace of the evening, but it didn't immediately scream of mortality.

I drank some water. I paced the floor of the farmhouse. I tried to focus on anything else, hoping the heavy feeling would simply pass through my system. But instead of fading, the sensation deepened, sinking its roots into my chest. First was gas, vomit, and then diarrhea – and that insidious pain in my chest.

As the hour crept toward ten o'clock, and then eleven, the ache morphed. It was no longer a dull irritation; it was becoming a heavy density, a thick, suffocating weight pressing down on my sternum. I went to the kitchen, splashed cold water on my face, and then to the bathroom and stared at my reflection in the mirror. My skin looked pale, slightly clammy.

Just a bad bug, I told the reflection. *It will pass.*

But it didn't pass. By midnight, the deception was unraveling. The pain had begun to radiate, a dull, electric throbbing that seemed to move independently of my breathing. The tightness in my chest was restricting the expansion of my lungs. Every breath required conscious, deliberate effort.

I sat on the edge of the bed in the dark, the silence of the farmhouse suddenly feeling oppressive rather than comforting. The physical pain was mounting, but a new, cold terror was beginning to rise alongside it.

I knew my own body. I had lived in it, pushed it, and relied on it for decades. What I was feeling was not a stomachache. It was not indigestion. It was something deeply, structurally wrong inside my chest. The invisible mule had pulled back its leg and was pressing its hoof directly center-mass against my heart, preparing to strike.

My mind raced. A torrent of thoughts flooded my consciousness, crashing against the shores of my meticulous, organized life. If this were a heart attack, where were the shooting pains down my left arm? Where was the dizziness? I was still conscious, still moving, still able to think. I looked for my Kardia device only to find it with a dead battery.

And then, the singular, overwhelming priority shattered every other thought: *Taylor.*

If I collapse right here, in the middle of the night, what happens to her? Who will find her? Who will explain to her why I am not getting up? The absolute horror of her waking up to find me incapacitated or dead on the floor of the farmhouse was more agonizing than the crushing weight in my chest.

That thought alone injected a surge of adrenaline into my system. I could not die here. I could not leave her alone in the dark.

The realization crystallized in my mind like freezing water. I was having a major cardiovascular event. I was forty miles from the nearest hospital equipped to handle a cardiac emergency. It was past midnight, cold and wet outside, and my daughter was sound asleep in the other room.

The pain flared, a warning shot from my failing heart. *Tick tock.*

The deception was over. The fight for my life—and to protect Taylor's—had just begun.

Chapter 2: The Priority of Care

For the first few hours, the battle was entirely psychological. It was me against my own anatomy, bargaining with a pain that refused to negotiate. As I paced the farmhouse from room to room, the discomfort evolved into a cruel, unyielding tightness. It was as if a heavy strap had been wrapped around my back and cinched tight across my chest, with every beat of my heart pulling the strap tighter.

I tried everything. I drank water. I chewed antacids. I contorted my body into stretches, hoping something would pop or align. I curled up on the floor, my knees drawn up in a desperate attempt to find a position that didn't feel like drowning in plain air. I knelt beside the bed, lay flat on the floor, and moved every joint I could move. Nothing worked.

As I moved through the house in the dark, my thoughts kept drifting back to earlier that day. What a stark contrast this agony was to the bright, clear blue skies we had enjoyed driving into Dallas. Those trips were essential to us—to our happiness and our routine. We listened to music, shopped for gourmet groceries, enjoyed a wonderful lunch, and taken Taylor to see a new OB/GYN doctor. I had even taken a thirty-minute phone call in the busy box store from a former corporate colleague, where I was the encouragement to him.

We talked about the crushing stress of our industry. We discussed the corporate mantra that had driven our lives: *"Do more with less."* The expectation is to constantly improve output despite dwindling resources. I had urged my friend to prioritize his health, to make decisions based on wellness instead of climbing a ladder that demanded endless sacrifice. The irony burned as fiercely as the pressure in my chest. Earlier that day, the doctors had meticulously evaluated Taylor, and true to form, she was perfectly healthy. I had mingled with medical staff, chatted with friends, and yet not one person had looked at me and said, "Henry, are you okay? You don't look well."

Because the signs of systemic stress—the kind that quietly ruins an executive's cardiovascular system—are entirely invisible until the mule rears back to kick.

As midnight dragged into the early morning hours, the undeniable reality settled over me: I needed medical intervention, and I needed it soon. But the simple solution of dialing 911 was, for me, a labyrinth of terrifying variables.

In rural East Texas, calling emergency services does not guarantee swift salvation. I had heard too many unsettling accounts of EMS taking up to two hours to navigate the backroads before finally arriving at a farmhouse. The thought of being trapped in this escalating agony for two more hours was almost more than my strained heart could bear.

But even if they arrived quickly, the question of EMS immediately brought me back to my singular, overriding priority: *Taylor.*

If an ambulance arrived with sirens blaring in the middle of the night, what would they do with her? She was sleeping peacefully just down the hall, blissfully unbothered by my relentless pacing. If I was loaded onto a stretcher, would the paramedics wake her up and take her with me into the chaotic, terrifying environment of an emergency room? Or, even more unthinkably, would they require me to leave her behind in an empty house to seek the care I desperately needed alone?

I could not put her through that trauma. My duty as a caregiver was a stubborn, ingrained instinct that outshone my own survival instinct.

Therefore, I had to save myself.

I reasoned that the rural highways to Mt. Pleasant would be better than the roads to Texarkana and that Hwy 259 would be mostly empty at this hour. I could drive myself. If the absolute worst happened and my heart gave out, causing me to crash, I would be on the main lane or shoulder where my truck would be visible to passing traffic. It was a morbid calculation, but it was the only one that preserved Taylor's peace.

By 3:00 AM, the situation was nearing a breaking point. Every breath felt like inhaling crushed glass. The urgency to leave was overwhelming, yet the one remaining complication paralyzed me—who would watch Taylor?

I pulled out my phone, my hands shaking slightly, and called a neighbor who lived about ten miles away. It was a tremendous risk calling someone so late, hoping the ringtone would break through their sleep. Mercifully, she answered. My voice was tight as I explained what was happening. Her response was immediate; she promised to get dressed and come straight over.

Ten minutes, I told myself. *Just hold on for ten more minutes.*

Knowing help was on the way for Taylor freed me to finally focus on my own survival. I grabbed my keys, stumbled out the door into the darkness, and started my truck. I backed it partially down the driveway and parked, leaving the engine running and the door open. I stood on the front steps, staring down the road, willing headlights to appear. The rumbling of the engine seemed to vibrate against my aching chest. Time, which is usually a constant, warped into something syrupy and unbearably slow.

When my neighbor's truck finally crunched onto the gravel, I felt a fraction of the weight lift. I gave her a breathless, rapid-fire explanation of my condition and the immediate instructions for Taylor. I told her I was going to Mt. Pleasant and that if I could not return, she could call every phone number in my action plan book until someone on the list would agree to come get Taylor.

This was the most desperate thought and action I have ever had to take regarding Taylor and the truth regarding my mortality.

Once Chris stepped inside the house, the tether was cut. There was nothing left to hold me back.

I climbed into the truck and shifted into gear as I slammed my foot on the accelerator. Anxiety and adrenaline, a potent and dangerous cocktail for a failing heart, surged through my veins. The isolation of the dark East Texas highway swallowed the truck as I sped toward the hospital, forty miles away.

The speedometer climbed. The darkness rushing past the windows was mesmerizing. In my heightened state of panic, I was entirely focused on the yellow lines illuminating under my headlights, desperate to reach the sterile haven of the Emergency Room.

Then, fate decided to display a sense of humor so cruel and absurd it defied comprehension.

I was traveling at seventy-four miles per hour. Out of the deep, black void of the rural roadside, a shape materialized a fraction of a second before the impact.

Smash.

The collision was violent and instantaneous. The sound of a heavy, brutal thud sent a terrifying shockwave directly through the steering wheel into my fragile chest. A deer had sprinted directly into my path. The force of the 74-mph impact threw the animal's body entirely over the cab of my truck.

My foot instinctively slammed on the brakes. As the truck lurched, my mind awash in a bizarre cocktail of disbelief and sheer terror. *Is this truly how my life ends?* To survive the onset of a massive heart attack for six hours in a lonely farmhouse, only to die on the side of a highway with a crushed front end from a deer?

For a singular, mad second, the caregiver in me hesitated. Should I stop and get out? Should I check on the animal? Do I need to dispatch the wounded animal?

But the dull, terrifying pain in my chest screamed louder than any empathy for the deer. Instinct swiftly murdered hesitation. The truck was still running. A quick glance at the dashboard confirmed the vitals: water temperature, oil pressure, and battery voltage were all within normal limits.

I took my foot off the brake and pressed down hard on the accelerator.

A short distance further, I merged onto the interstate, the urgency overtook reality. The speedometer needle swept toward 90 miles per hour. I blew past hulking tractor-trailers in the dead of the night, locking my vision solely on the side of the highway looking for the next mile marker. I needed to see marker 162 as the number counted down from 178. The world outside the glass became a blurry tunnel. My only focus was maintaining control of a battered truck while the muscles in my chest screamed.

After what felt like a lifetime—thirty agonizing minutes of high-speed terror—the glowing red letters of the hospital's Emergency Room came into view. I threw the truck haphazardly into a parking space near the entrance, caring nothing for the lines.

I stumbled out of the cab into the wet night air. The stark fluorescent lights of the entrance guided me toward the glass doors. The dread was a physical weight now, heavier than the invisible strap on my chest. It wasn't just the exertion of driving a wrecked truck at 90 mph during an adrenaline spike; it was the unshakeable, profound fear of the medical reality that awaited me inside those automatic doors.

The deception was long gone. The real fight was about to begin.

Chapter 3: The Anatomy of a STEMI and The Widow Maker

To truly understand the gravity of the panic that unfolded in the ER that early December morning, it is vital to step away from the adrenaline-fueled timeline and examine exactly what was happening—silently and devastatingly—inside my chest.

When a patient arrives at a hospital complaining of chest pain, medical staff immediately performs an electrocardiogram (EKG) to monitor the heart's electrical activity. What they are looking for is a specific, terrifying spike on that paper printout. The doctors in my emergency room saw exactly that. I was suffering from what the medical community calls STEMI.

STEMI stands for **ST-Elevation Myocardial Infarction**.

To break that down: an "infarction" means tissue death due to a lack of blood supply, causing damage to the myocardium (the heart muscle). The "ST-Elevation" refers to the specific EKG anomaly, indicating that the damage is occurring at that moment. A STEMI is not a mild warning sign, a partial narrowing, or a temporary spasm. It is the most severe, catastrophic type of heart attack a human body can endure. It occurs when a major coronary artery is abruptly and entirely blocked, usually by a ruptured plaque that triggers a massive blood clot.

In my case, the total blockage occurred in the most dangerous possible location: the Left Anterior Descending artery. In the medical world, a 100% blockage of the LAD is ominously known by a grim nickname: **The Widow Maker**.

To understand why this specific artery carries such a morbid title, you must understand the plumbing of the heart. The Left Anterior Descending artery is the main pipeline of the cardiovascular system. It runs straight down the front of the heart and is responsible for supplying almost half of the blood volume to the left ventricle—the main pumping chamber that pushes oxygenated blood to the rest of the body. When the LAD is choked off completely, the heart is starved of a massive amount of oxygen. The muscle tissue begins to die rapidly. Without immediate medical intervention, a Widow Maker almost always leads to sudden cardiac arrest.

The nickname itself originated decades ago, during a time when severe cardiovascular disease was historically considered a danger to middle-aged and older men primarily. Because men were statistically more likely at the time to suffer from massive, sudden heart attacks, the near-total blockage of the LAD became a dark, colloquial shorthand among doctors and nurses for a fatal event that would abruptly leave a man's wife a widow.

Today, modern cardiology acknowledges that the term "Widow Maker" is somewhat outdated and misleading, as this catastrophic blockage violently affects both men and women. The danger does not discriminate by gender. However, the sheer lethality of the name remains entirely accurate. It signifies a cardiac crisis where the margin for error is nonexistent.

In the medical community, there is a fundamental rule regarding a STEMI Widow Maker: *Time is muscle.*

Every passing minute that the Left Anterior Descending artery remains blocked, more of the heart wall permanently dies. The gold standard for treating a STEMI is to get the patient into a cardiac catheterization lab and open the blocked artery within ninety minutes of the initial symptom onset.

As I lay in the ER, watching the frantic preparations around me, the horrifying reality of my timeline crystallized. The dull ache at the farmhouse had started at 9:15 PM. By the time I arrived at the hospital, it was nearing dawn the next day. The clock had been ticking relentlessly the entire time I had been pacing the farmhouse floor, negotiating with the pain, calling my neighbor, and flying down the highway at 90 miles per hour after hitting a deer.

I had not waited ninety minutes. I had spent nearly 7.5 hours walking around with a 100% blocked Widow Maker.

I had survived the impossible, but my heart was severely damaged. The deception of pain had nearly cost me everything, and the true, brutal battle to physically clear the blockage and halt the dying muscle was about to begin on the operating table.

Chapter 4: The Widow Maker

The interior of the Emergency Room was a stark, jarring contrast to the chaotic terror of the highway. After hurling myself through the glass doors, my heart pounding a panicked rhythm against the crushing weight in my chest, I was met with absolute silence. The lobby was entirely empty. Not a single person could be seen or heard.

I leaned heavily against the front desk, my breathing shallow and ragged. I knocked on the closed doors. I called out for assistance. My voice echoed uselessly against the sterile walls. The delay felt insurmountable. Every second I stood there was a second that the invisible mule continued to press its terrible weight into my sternum.

Tick tock.

Finally, after about five agonizing minutes, and a strong kick to the locked door, a young nurse appeared from down the hall.

"I believe I am having a heart attack," I managed to say. The words felt surreal, hanging in the bright, fluorescent air between us.

Immediately, the sluggishness of the empty lobby evaporated. She called for the triage nurse. They swooped in, a blur of motion taking measurements, asking rapid-fire questions, and listening to my breathless answers. Within moments, I was being rushed down a long hallway to meet a much larger team of nurses and doctors waiting for me.

It was there, lying amidst the sudden flurry of medical personnel, that a doctor approached me, and I heard the word for the very first time.

STEMI.

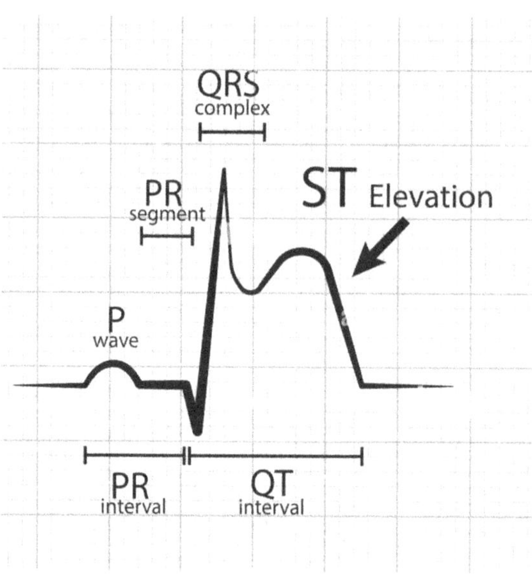

The doctor spoke the acronym to the surrounding team, and the sharp, unfamiliar sound of it stuck with me. He leaned over and confirmed the diagnosis without sugarcoating the severity. I was experiencing a severe ST-Elevation Myocardial Infarction. The blockage in my Left Anterior Descending artery meant my heart was rapidly dying. I was facing the Widow Maker head-on.

The crushing weight of the diagnosis mirrored the very physical agony I had been enduring for hours. I had waited entirely too long before driving to the hospital. Looking back, the realization of that delay shifted from unwise to perilous. The clock had been relentlessly ticking, burning through the precious window of time where heart muscle can be saved, the entire time I had been pacing the farmhouse floor, negotiating with pain.

As the medical team hustled around me, prepping me for the cardiac catheterization lab to save my life, the adrenaline in my system mixed equally with fear and determination. The stark reality of the night had fully settled over me. This wasn't an inconvenience or a bad case of indigestion. This was a life-altering threshold, forcing me to confront my own extreme fragility.

Yet, even as they waited for the on-call doctors to make their way to the hospital, I laid there underneath the brim of my favorite cowboy hat. Later, the nurses moved me to prepare me for the operating table, all the while my mind remained anchored to a reality far away from the hospital. *Taylor.*

They wheeled me into the sterile, brilliantly lit operating room. The bright surgical lights directly overhead were blocked by my hat. From under the brim, I saw a hand reach for my hat to which I said no! In Texas, don't mess with a man's horse or his hat. To which the nurse responded, my hospital my rules, you can keep that hat, but I am taking your pants – and she did! The quiet hum of complex medical machinery filled the room. The cardiologist and the nurses discussed the state of my heart with a calm, practiced focus that was almost dizzying. As I lay there on the table, completely exposed, watching the monitors display the sluggish movement of blood through my own failing heart, I felt profoundly vulnerable.

But I refused to be helpless.

Pain medication was conspicuously absent from my IV. No morphine coursed through my veins to dull the agony in my chest or hinder my ability to think.

That was not an oversight. It was my choice.

The medical staff was entirely focused on the crisis happening inside my chest. To them, I was a critical cardiac patient requiring immediate revascularization. But to me, I was still Taylor's caregiver. The fear that consumed me on that table wasn't just the fear of a scalpel, a catheter, or dying. My terror stemmed from one harrowing, consuming scenario: I had no time to inform Taylor about what was happening, or why I wouldn't be home when she woke up in the morning.

No one in the room seemed to acknowledge my urgent, desperate wish to remain alert and aware. I refused the pain medication so my mind would stay sharp. I needed to be able to communicate. If my heart gave out on that table, if things went irreparably wrong, I had to be lucid enough to tell someone—*anyone*—how to access the crucial documents, the legal plans, and the resources I had meticulously arranged back home. I needed them to know where the go-kits and notebooks were, complete with their labels and tabs, all waiting in duplicate form. I needed to be able to unlock my phone with the critical contacts that would be needed.

For two and a half hours, I lay on that table, completely alert, feeling the pressure and presence of the tools working inside my body. My mind was an endless, high-speed dialogue of fear, regret for waiting so long, and desperate hope.

Finally, the cardiologist successfully placed three stents to force the Widow Maker open and restore the flow of life-saving oxygen to the starved muscle of my heart. A fourth stent, they explained, would be necessary, but it had to wait for another day. It would be required before I could be discharged.

By the time the procedure ended, approximately seven and a half hours had elapsed since the pain first started in the farmhouse. Seven and a half hours with a 100% blocked LAD.

The immediate crisis was over. The stents were holding the artery open. But as they transported me to the Intensive Care Unit for monitoring, the silence of the hospital closed in around me once again. I was alive, miraculously so, but the damage was done. I would soon learn that it would take ninety agonizing days to comprehend the full extent of the permanent injury to my heart.

The Widow Maker had taken its best shot. I survived the night. But as I closed my eyes in the ICU, the true weight of the recovery ahead—and the second chance God had inexplicably granted me—was only just beginning to dawn on me.

Chapter 5: The Stents and the ICU

Surviving the initial strike of a Widow Maker heart attack is a miracle in itself, but the battle does not abruptly end when the catheter is removed. Instead, you are wheeled into the Intensive Care Unit, stripped of your autonomy, and tethered to a dozen different machines that beep and hum, monitoring the fragile rhythm of your second chance at life. For eighty-eight hours, the ICU became my world—a sterile, timeless medical prison where day and night blurred together under constant fluorescent lighting.

The immediate aftermath of the surgery left me physically wrecked. Although the three stents had restored the blood flow through the Left Anterior Descending artery, my body had endured massive trauma. I had spent seven and a half hours with a one-hundred-percent blockage. The heart muscle had been starved, stretched, and tortured. Now that the flow had been restored, my body had reacted with severe fluid retention. Over those few days, the ICU pumped my system full of medications and fluids, causing me to gain over twenty pounds of sheer water weight.

It was a suffocating sensation. Lying in that hospital bed, I literally felt like I was drowning from the inside out. My leg was already bruised and aching from the surgery, but the added pressure of the fluid made every single breath a conscious, exhausting labor. I hated the feeling of being trapped in a body that felt swollen and foreign.

Yet, despite the physical misery, the ICU was the place where the profound spiritual reality of what had just happened truly settled over me.

When you find yourself on death's doorstep, stripped of your strength, your meticulously planned routines, and your identity as a capable caregiver, you are left alone with the absolute core of who you are. In those quiet, terrifying hours in the ICU, surrounded by the mechanical breathing of machines, I turned to prayer.

But it wasn't a desperate, panicked prayer of a stranger begging for a favor. As I closed my eyes against the harsh hospital lights, I found immense comfort in the realization that I did not have to introduce myself to God. He knows me, and I know Him. Our conversations in that room were easy, peaceful, and deeply intimate, primarily because it wasn't a first date. I had walked with Him for years, leaning on His understanding when I couldn't find my own. I lay there and thanked Him, not just for the skilled hands of the cardiologist, but for the profound grace that allowed me to survive an entirely blocked Widow Maker after driving myself forty miles at ninety miles an hour.

Still, my peace was continuously interrupted by my unrelenting concern for Taylor.

I was confined to the bed, physically unable to fulfill my role as her caregiver, but my mind never stopped strategizing. I had to advocate for myself, pushing through the exhaustion to communicate with the medical staff, because I needed to get out of that bed and get back to her. I quickly realized that even on death's doorstep, you must be your own advocate, or else things simply won't happen fast enough. I used every ounce of corporate communication training I had ever received to tell the nurses and doctors who was in charge and exactly how things were going to get done regarding my recovery plan.

On Friday, December 19th, the doctors returned to finish the job. The initial crisis had been stabilized by the first three stents, but a fourth stent was required to fully prop open the damaged artery and secure the passage. It was a condition that had to be met before they would even consider discharging me.

Going back onto the operating table for the fourth stent was mentally taxing. The adrenaline of the initial emergency had completely faded, replaced by deep, bone-weary fatigue. But I focused on the singular goal: getting home to Taylor. I watched the monitors again, enduring the procedure, knowing that this small piece of metal was the final key to unlocking the ICU door.

By Friday evening, with the fourth stent successfully in place, and the heart pump that was initially installed to assist my weakened heart now removed, the conversations shifted from critical stabilization to discharge planning. The doctors were amazed by my vitals, given the severity of the blockage. I was alive, and the hardware was holding. But they were quick to temper my eagerness to leave with a stark dose of reality. The immediate danger had passed, but my heart was profoundly damaged. It would take ninety days before they could perform an echocardiogram to accurately map the scarred tissue and determine exactly how much capacity my broken heart had remaining.

I decided that I was going to be released the following day, Saturday, December 20th, but I was not walking out of that hospital as a free man. I was trading the ICU monitors for a different kind of tether.

Before they would sign the discharge papers, the doctors presented me with a strict set of conditions and a piece of equipment that would become the bane of my existence for the next several weeks: a wearable defibrillator.

It was a heavy, complicated vest designed to shock my heart back into rhythm if it suddenly stopped. They insisted it was necessary, a vital bridge of protection while my heart was in its most vulnerable state of healing. I grimly strapped the bulky hardware around my chest, adjusting the sensors against my shaved skin.

I called it my "little helper." It was a sarcastic moniker for a device that I immediately detested. But if wearing it was the only way they would let me walk out of those doors and get back to the farmhouse—and back to Taylor—then I was prepared to wear it into battle.

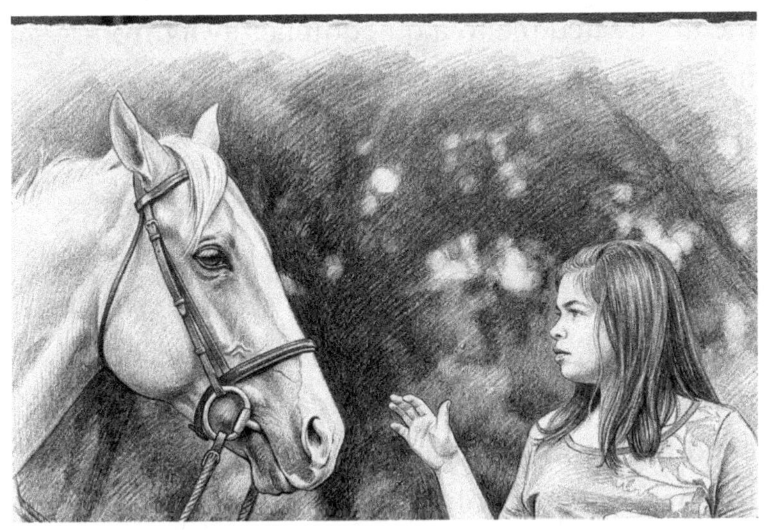

Chapter 6: Discharge and the Little Helper

The irony of modern medicine is that doctors will save your life in a high-tech operating room, but they cannot truly heal the mind from the trauma it has just endured. When Saturday, December 20th, finally arrived, I was eager beyond words to rip myself away from the monitors and the sterile walls. My brother, Wes, arrived to assist in my great escape from the medical prison. He picked me up, treated me to a quiet dinner away from hospital food, and then drove us toward my recovery.

Yet, stepping out of the hospital was not the victorious, liberating experience I had envisioned. I felt frail. I was exhausted. And securely strapped beneath my shirt was the Life Vest—my "little helper" that the hospital had mandated as a condition of my release. The heavy device felt less like an insurance policy and more like a constant, physical reminder that I was still in critical condition, walking around with a heart that couldn't fully be trusted.

When we finally returned home to the farmhouse, I assumed the familiar walls would bring an instant sense of peace. I was wrong. The first profound psychological hurdle of my recovery was entirely unexpected, and it began the moment I went to lie back down on that first night at home.

I crawled into the very same bed where the event had begun just days prior. It had never occurred to me how heavily that specific space held the terrible memories of the longest night of my life. As the darkness settled over the house, the quiet peace I used to love was entirely shattered by my own racing thoughts.

The following day we all packed for Taylor and me to relocate to the Dallas area. Once there and for three more nights in a row, lying in bed, I relived the entire episode minute by agonizing minute. The dull ache, the realization, the pacing, the adrenaline, the deer crashing into the truck. The thoughts played on a terrifying, endless loop. The confusion I had felt that night was slowly being replaced by a lingering anger. I survived, yes, but my life moving forward was forever marred by the fact that my body had betrayed me.

I realized very quickly that recovering in absolute rural isolation, and hours away from major medical centers and Taylor's beloved Aspire Day Hab, was going to breed anxiety rather than healing.

We had made a strategic decision to relocate temporarily even before discharge from the hospital. We packed up and began what I called "hotel camping" in The Colony. It kept us close to Dallas, close to the doctors, and most importantly, close to our incredible network of friends and family.

That first week in the city, the true spirit of friendship revealed itself in ways that left me deeply, fiercely humbled. The transition could not have happened without our people stepping up to fill the massive gap my weakened state had created.

Richard welcomed us to share Christmas lunch with his family, refusing to let us celebrate the holiday alone in a hotel room. Luis constantly checked in, running supplies and taking me out to dinner just to get me out of the room. Chuck graciously ferried the necessary items up from the farm. Fred played shuttle driver perfectly, getting Taylor where she needed to go.

Marie, Wes, and Sharon helped us get settled and organized in the hotel room, so it didn't feel quite so chaotic. Margaret effortlessly took over shuttling Taylor to her day hab in Lewisville, where Taylor happily bounced through the doors into a crowd calling her name. Marie stepped into a central caregiving role for us, and Chris proved to be an amazing steward of the farm and Suny while we were stranded in the city. Julie and Steve provided respite over the first weekend so that I could rest.

After 30 hours, having settled into the hotel, I resumed the role of Taylor's primary caregiver. I desperately needed support myself, yet I was back on duty both day and night for Taylor. By the fourth night, I realized this situation was precariously dangerous. But what options did I have?

Without this incredible circle of family and friends, those early days of recovery would not have just been difficult; they would have been impossible. They formed a safety net underneath me while I attempted to navigate my fragile new reality.

My brother Wes had helped me escape the hospital, but my friends were helping me survive the aftermath.

My primary focus during those hotel days was simply to increase my strength and improve my shallow breathing. The only thing worse than the pain of the heart attack was the sensation of drowning from the inside out of my lungs. Eventually, the fluid retention from the ICU slowly began to dissipate, and I lost twenty-six pounds in the 14 days following the attack. I was struggling to establish an appetite, finding that breakfast was the only meal I could truly tolerate. But my mind was stable, aided immensely by 'Doc,' who helped me understand exactly how powerful the mind's operating system is, and how it employed these stages of grief to process the trauma of the Widow Maker.

But the most difficult struggle during those early weeks wasn't the breathing, the weight loss, or the cabin fever in the hotel. It was the Vest.

Learning how to sleep with the heavy defibrillator strapped to my chest was a misery. It was physically uncomfortable, but the technological flaws were even worse. On more than one terrifying morning, the defibrillator system triggered. The alarms began sounding, warning me that it was preparing to deliver a massive shock to my chest. Complete panic gripped me until I was able to stop the machine, canceling the trigger before the 1500-pound mule could kick me all over again.

I was constantly fidgeting with the sensors, a nervous habit powered by a deep-seated anxiety that I was doing something wrong, or that it would misfire. As I jokingly told my friends, I would have failed miserably at being a terrorist because I couldn't stop messing with my detonator.

If my prayer in the ICU was one of thanksgiving for survival, my prayer in the hotel room was singular and exhausting: *Lord, let me see this Life Vest as a helper, and not as a terrifying countdown clock.*

Chapter 7: The Weight of the Vest (Weeks 1-4)

By the time three full weeks had passed since my discharge, the hotel camping in The Colony had served its purpose. My body was slowly reacquainting itself with the basic rhythms of life. Though my appetite remained small—breakfast being the primary meal I could tolerate—my sleep began to arrive in more solid, three-hour blocks. I was walking up to three miles a day, and my mind felt sharp enough to spend small chunks of time working on the computer. My friends were still actively hovering, bringing this and that to keep Taylor and me functional and in clean clothes. I was profoundly grateful, yet a deep, undeniable pull was growing in my chest.

I was longing for the farm. I needed to see the open sky of East Texas. I needed to breathe without the faint trace of city smog in my lungs. My metallic taste from the medical prison was dissipating, and I was eager for the familiar quiet of rural living. More than anything, I needed to prove to myself that I could return to our sanctuary without the terrifying memories of the event entirely overpowering the peace over the land.

With our friend Fred graciously driving, we made our first foray out of the city and back toward Mt.

Pleasant to attend my first follow-up visit with the cardiologist. The drive itself felt like a crossing of thresholds. A short checkup with the cardiologist in Mt. Pleasant, followed by a drive back home along the same route I had taken to the hospital, ensued. We stopped at a local bank for cash, grabbed Taylor's medications at the pharmacy, and walked through Spring Market to pick up simple groceries. The stark, comforting difference between these small-town stores and the grandiose, fast-paced intensity of the city was striking. It grounded me.

The cardiologist's appointment offered a dose of pragmatic reality. My weight hovered at 185 pounds—down significantly from my 217 pounds at discharge. While my heart was functioning, it was still healing, and I was strictly bound to my "helper," the Life Vest, for at least ninety more days until a follow-up echocardiogram could determine my heart's remaining capacity.

The doctor's advice for my daily activity was surprisingly simple, though profound in its implications: *You are okay to do whatever you want as long as you can breathe, stay conscious, and talk while doing it. If you can't, then stop.*

When we finally returned to the farm, accompanied by Chris, the air was crisp, and the familiar sights of the pasture were a balm to my spirit. But the reality of my physical limitations became immediately, undeniably clear, particularly when it collided with my deeply ingrained, OCD-driven desire for order.

Before the Widow Maker, I managed the farmhouse at top speed. A piece of dust, a chore out of place, an uneven arrangement, it was all handled with endless energy. Now, I discovered just how intensely demanding being OCD actually was. I would start cleaning, turning, lifting, wiping, and within minutes, my body would harshly demand a pause. I was forced to sit and explicitly rest between every minor task. The sheer exhaustion forced a painful compromise: I had to accept things being out of place or burn precious energy that should have been spent walking or healing. It was a rigorous, daily negotiation that humbled me constantly.

As the days passed and the first four weeks since the event culminated, we settled into a hybrid routine. Chet, Linda, and Chris were constant fixtures, stepping in to tackle projects around the farm, offering fellowship that anchored Taylor and me to a sense of community. I found a fragile balance between resting, working, capturing sunrise photography, and simply sitting at the pavilion, listening to the birds, the wind chimes, and the wildlife.

Yet, healing was not linear. The nights remained difficult. As I lay in the quiet, the traumatic remnants of the event continued to surface. My mind relentlessly revealed its startling capacity to remember, replay, and relate the experience of that terrible night. Every time my heart fluttered, every time my pulse quickened, the hyper-vigilance would grip me: *Is it happening again?*

When a bitter Texas ice storm, what we called "ice-a-geddon"—rolled across the farm, the cold air seemed to physically suck the remaining energy directly out of my chest. Walking out to feed the cow or crack the ice on Suny's water tank was necessary, and ironically, I felt fine, but my little helper continued to trigger false alarms. But even amidst the freezing temperatures and the intrusive anxieties, there was a profound undercurrent of clarity.

During those first four weeks, wrapped in winter's chill and strapped into a burdensome vest, I arrived at a place of unshakeable peace. I had genuinely believed on December 16th that my time to leave this earth had arrived. Staring death in the face fundamentally reorganized my perspective. I recalled the quiet, painless peace that had overwhelmed me in the hospital, the grace that enveloped me even as I watched doctors manually restoring blood flow to my dying heart.

I accepted that I emerged with an impaired body. The heavy vest strapped to my chest was a testament to that. But in exchange, my spirit was infinitely lighter. I possessed a crystalline understanding of my purpose—to continue as a caregiver for Taylor, to photograph the elusive perfect sunrise, to share laughter with friends, and to live this second chance with immense intentionality. The future remained a mystery, but as week four drew to a close, I was joyfully taking the discovery of this new life one single minute at a time.

Chapter 8: Breaking Free (Weeks 5-8)

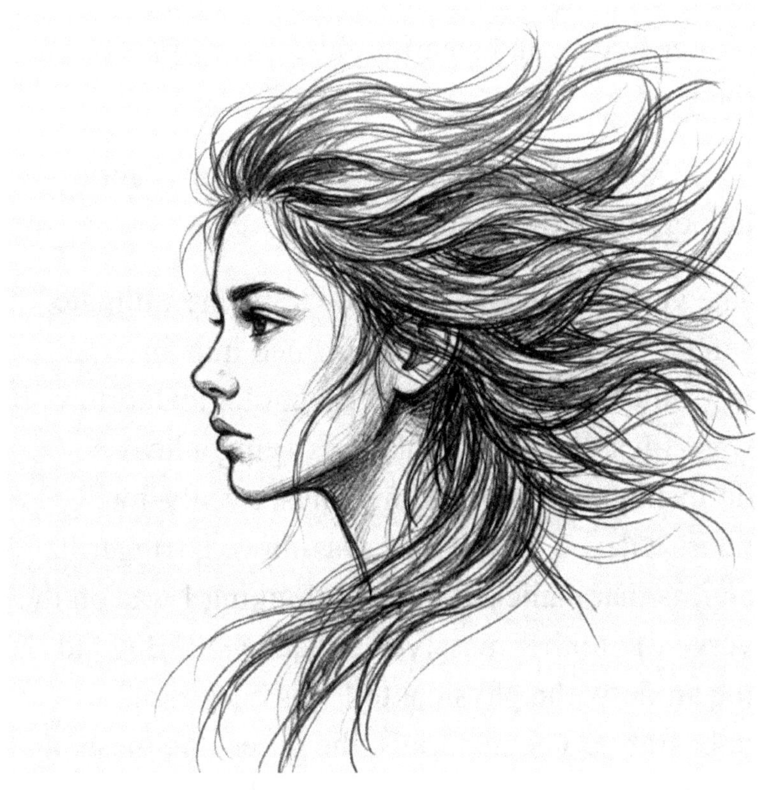

Recovery is rarely a steady incline; it often feels like a series of fierce negotiations with your own body. By the time six weeks had passed since my brother Wes first drove me away from the hospital, those negotiations were becoming increasingly frustrating. Physically, I was growing stronger.

The deep, heavy exhaustion that accompanied every movement was lifting. I was actively feeding the cow, breaking ice on hay bales during the winter freeze, and clearing fallen tree limbs out in the yard.

Yet, I was still physically tethered to my "little helper" the Life Vest.

The vest, which was designed to be my ultimate safety net, had slowly transformed into an instrument of physical and psychological torture. It wasn't just the sheer bulk of carrying a heavy defibrillator strapped to my chest twenty-four hours a day. The software was flawed, triggering alarms that panicked me into thinking I was on the verge of another massive cardiac event. Beyond the anxiety, the physical toll was becoming unbearable. The materials, the wires, the mesh, and the heavy sensors rubbing endlessly against my skin had caused painful lesions. I couldn't sleep. I was constantly fidgeting with the device, haunted by the fear that my nervous adjustments were somehow doing more damage to my healing heart.

A breaking point was inevitable.

It happened about midnight. I was lying in bed, exhausted but too uncomfortable and anxious to sleep, wrestling with the wires and the mesh. Finally, a sense of clarity pierced through the frustration. I realized that the chronic stress and severe sleep deprivation caused by the vest were actively hindering my recovery. If I was going to heal, I needed rest. So, feeling slightly rebellious but entirely resolute, I reached over, unhooked the device, and completely removed the battery.

I set it aside, lay my head on the pillow, and experienced the best, most profound sleep I'd had since the night of December 16th.

It took immense courage to trust my body again without a machine monitoring it, but the relief was instantaneous. Almost overnight, my anxiety dissipated. I was sleeping deeply, relaxing fully, and feeling human once more.

With the heavy burden of the vest lifted, a renewed sense of freedom washed over us. Before the Widow Maker, Taylor and I had been dreaming of a road trip through Central Texas. Realizing there was no better time to reclaim our lives than the present, we packed up the truck and hit the open road.

We embarked on a 900-mile journey through the Texas Hill Country. We drove through Athens, wound our way down toward Austin, taking in the expansive skies and rolling landscapes before heading north to Dallas. It was a trip filled with rest, phenomenal food, and time spent with incredible friends and making new ones along the way. A major highlight was taking Taylor to visit her crew at Aspire Day Hab in Lewisville. Walking through those doors felt like walking onto the set of *Cheers*; the entire room erupted, shouting "Taylor!!!!!!!" as she bounced joyfully through the crowd, beaming from ear to ear. Watching her be so celebrated was medicine for my soul.

The culmination of that 900-mile road trip was an appointment with a new doctor in Frisco. It had become abundantly clear that there was a massive disparity between city doctors and rural medical services, and I needed an expert who was willing to truly partner with me in my recovery.

It was during this visit that my suspicions were completely validated: I wasn't crazy. My wearable defibrillator had, in fact, been defective. Hearing a medical professional confirm that the software was inaccurate and the physical lesions were unacceptable was an incredibly vindicating moment.

The Frisco doctor gave me a referral to a new, highly rated cardiologist, scheduling a comprehensive suite of blood and urine tests and a fresh echocardiogram for the following week. This was exactly what I wanted—actual science and hard metrics to tell me precisely how my broken heart was healing. Based on my recent physical activity, such as hauling limbs in the yard, driving the tractor, hoeing the high tunnels, and caring for Taylor, it was clear my heart was handling a reasonable workload. It certainly felt more engaging and productive than walking on a treadmill or pedaling a stationary bike at the local cardiac rehab facility—an offer I had politely laughed at and declined.

However, leaving the vest behind didn't mean abandoning responsibility. By the time I reached the seven-week mark—forty-nine days since discharge—I made a solemn promise to myself and to Taylor. I would not take the tremendous grace God had shown me for granted.

I despised the handful of medications I had to swallow each morning, but I took them exactly as prescribed. As the weather warmed and the urge to tackle major spring projects around the farm grew intensely, I forced myself to be smart. I prioritized wellness over stubbornness. I maintained a strict, heart-healthy diet and guarded my sleep schedules fiercely. My vast network of friends served as a chorus of accountability, urging me to be responsible and faithful to the healing process. I recognized their warnings for what they were: the purest expression of love. Responding to that love meant doing what was right and staying accountable.

My mind was finally beginning to look forward rather than backward. Sitting quietly at the farm, untethered from the machine and feeling the brisk air in my lungs, the future began to look expansive again. On my desk sat a white paper outlining our next dream: an RV road trip out to the rugged Texas Big Bend country, and eventually, an extended journey to the western high country and monument area.

For the first time since the Widow Maker, I wasn't just surviving. I was planning to live.

Chapter 9: A Second Chance at Life (Weeks 9-12)

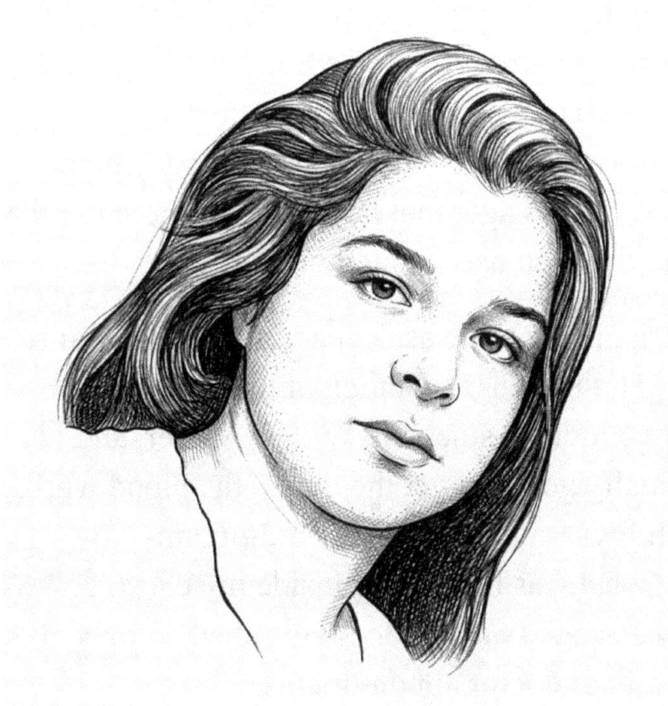

By week nine, the frantic, survival-oriented energy of the first two months had given way to a quieter, more profound era of recovery. Over the past sixty-three days, I had absorbed a lifetime's worth of education on cardiovascular function, maintenance, and nutritional chemistry. More importantly, I had developed a vast, unshakable appreciation for my friends, my family, and the resilient mechanics of my own body.

Heading back into the city for a battery of tests felt different this time. As Taylor and I loaded up the truck on a Tuesday morning, a distinct sense of déjà vu washed over me. It was a Tuesday night, all those weeks ago, that had quietly ushered in the second life God had granted me.

This trip, however, wasn't characterized by fear. I felt a genuine sense of anticipation. It had been over two months since the Widow Maker, and I was finally going to get the data—the blood work, a fresh EKG, and a new echocardiogram—to reveal what was happening inside my chest. I gladly arranged our Wednesday schedule to be a marathon of doctor appointments.

The results were, simply put, astounding.

My primary care physician relayed blood chemistry first. Everything looked fantastic. My triglycerides were very low, indicating an excellent ratio. The doctor’s "treatment" plan for a slightly low HDL? Eat more walnuts. That meant I was definitely going to have to be nicer to my friends Richard and Karen, who always shared their wonderful harvests of nuts. The only slight abnormality was my glucose, which was elevated as a side effect of two of my strict heart medications.

But it was the meeting with my new cardiologist that provided the true miracle. He looked at the echo results—sixty-three days after a massive, 100% LAD blockage that absolutely should have killed me—and delivered the verdict. Functionally, my heart was operating on the "low side of normal." My ejection fraction was at 55%, and my overall circulation was superb.

The cardiologist looked at me and said, "The treatment plan is simple: Say 'God is good, 'realize this is what a miracle looks like, and thank everyone for their prayers."

Prayer works. The unexplainable peace I had felt in the ICU had manifested into a physical reality. My mission moving forward was clear. I needed to keep doing my self-guided rehab. I needed to learn to grow the foods that benefited my diet at the farm. And most importantly, I needed to pursue each day with an earnest desire to be generous towards others, to stay happy, and to deeply love the people around me.

Through all of this, my greatest silent supporter was sitting right next to me in the truck. I have always known that Taylor has far more capacity and intuition than typical assessments might suggest, but the prior two months proved it beyond a shadow of a doubt. I am convinced she somehow implicitly knew I was impaired. Without words, she adjusted. She helped me in numerous, subtle ways to get through each grueling day and night. Her angels were constantly present, guarding us both, and she had adapted to our new normal fantastically.

By week twelve—nearing the threshold of my first 90 days—our hybrid farm and city life had found its rhythm. The open road had become our second home. We completed another week-long journey around DFW and North Texas. The itinerary was simple but vital: dropping in on family, seeing friends like LeeAnna, Mark, Robert, Danny, Luis, and Sharon, and enjoying great food. Watching other people live life to the maximum inspired me to do the same.

During this trip, it felt like the final pieces of our medical puzzle fell into place. Taylor met her new neurologist, and I instantly liked the man. He asked what we had been doing and how it was going. When I explained our routine and noted that she was doing very well, he smiled and said, "I don't like changing something that works, so let's keep doing that."

My own appointments echoed that same, refreshing pragmatism. I sat with my new cardiologist for a forty-five-minute carotid ultrasound, watching the monitors as he scanned left and right. The verdict? The pipes were completely clear. There was nothing to treat with intervention, and no new medications to add.

This was a doctor who didn't just throw pharmaceuticals at a chart. My LDL was holding strong at 41 (well under the target of 55), and my vitals were stellar.

His parting instruction as I walked out of the clinic was the best piece of medical advice I’ve ever received: *"Go live a normal life."*

I felt an immense responsibility to pay that grace forward. It sparked a personal mantra that I carried back to the farm: Find a doctor you trust. Eat well and exercise. Tell your family and friends how much they mean to you. And wake up every single day with the singular goal to be happy and generous.

At thirteen weeks out from the Widow Maker, I was finally truly unburdened. The anxiety was gone. I was happy, relaxed, deeply grateful, and gloriously alive.

Conclusion

Day 100 arrived not with a rigid sense of finality, but with the expansive joy of the open road. As Easter approached, Taylor and I were traveling again, visiting family and friends. Celebrating the holiday on the road felt incredibly fitting. This year, the meaning of resurrection —of rising to a new life —was not just a theological concept—it was visceral. It was a second chance actively beating in my chest.

Looking back on the Widow Maker, the hospital stays, the unbearable Life Vest, and the anxiety of the first 100 days, the profound transformation wasn't solely physical. It was entirely spiritual.

As caregivers, we often operate under the exhausting illusion of control. We build detailed binders, label medical history files, and write instructions in duplicate. We try to legally and logistically secure a future in which we are absent. But the events of December 16th forced me to confront a harsh, unvarnished truth.

The reality is that our crisis will most likely appear suddenly and violently. And despite our most meticulous, desperate efforts to plan for every contingency, the devastating truth is that the next person to arrive will probably not have the desire, or the capacity, to rearrange their entire life to place our special person as their absolute priority in the exact way we have.

Things are going to be different. The meticulous schedules might falter. The daily nuances we have perfected through years of love might be lost in translation.

But within that terrifying realization, I found an immense, liberating grace. They will find a way to make it all work.

As a caregiver, you must realize that you cannot permanently control the future, no matter how hard you try. What you *can* do is pour everything you have into the present. While we are here, while we possess breath and strength, we must love them fiercely. We must give everything we can to provide our special people with the best, most vibrant life possible today. We take them on road trips. We introduce them to friends. We ensure they know, unequivocally, that they are celebrated and loved.

And then, we must let go. We must accept that what happens next is completely within the purview of our God.

Surviving the Widow Maker taught me that my life, and Taylor's life, rest in hands much larger than my own. If He can part the sudden, catastrophic blockage of a Widow Maker to grant me a second chance, He is more than capable of watching over the person I love most.

We must trust Him completely for ourselves, and just as importantly, we must trust Him completely for our loved ones.

The fear of the unknown no longer paralyzes me. I wake up each morning at the farmhouse with a remarkably simple, joyous mandate: Go live a normal life. Eat well. Tell your family and friends how much they mean to you. Wake up with the goal to be happy, and when you can, be exceptionally generous.

The future remains a mystery, but we are taking the discovery one glorious minute at a time.

The end

This song poured out of me on Easter morning of 2026. Being back home on the farm, almost 100 days after a heart attack nearly took everything from me, I was simply overwhelmed by the breathtaking gift of being alive. These words capture that exact moment of sheer joy and redemption.

https://suno.com/s/WToPumJQCupcLmKx

written by Henry Cross

Spectacular is Here! (Upbeat Celebration)

Spectacular is Here!

Verse 1

Throw the curtains wide and let the morning in,

I've got a second chance and I'm ready to begin!

The coffee's pouring hot, and the sky is painting blue,

Oh, what a crazy miracle, to wake up here with you.

Chorus

And the Maker's up there winking in the rising of the sun,

Saying, "Morning to you, child! Look at all we've just begun!"

So leave the heavy worries at the bottom of the stairs,

We've got a spectacular today, a gift beyond compare.

Yeah, I'm dancing in the daylight, I've got nothing left to fear,

Spectacular is waiting... Spectacular is here!

Verse 2

Well, the monitors were beeping, yeah, the road was getting rough,

But heaven pulled me back and said, “You haven’t loved enough!”

Now every little moment is a firecracker spark,

I'm throwing out the blueprints and I'm lighting up the dark.

Chorus

‘Cause the Maker’s up there winking in the rising of the sun,

Saying, “Morning to you, child! Look at all we’ve just begun!”

So leave the heavy worries at the bottom of the stairs,

We’ve got a spectacular today, a gift beyond compare.

Yeah, I’m dancing in the daylight, I’ve got nothing left to fear,

Spectacular is waiting... Spectacular is here!

Bridge

With Taylor smiling back at me, the rhythm's running sweet,

I'm kicking off the muddy boots and stepping to the beat.

I got a brand new lease on life, let the hallelujahs spin,

When you face the widow maker, you just celebrate the win!

Chorus

'Cause the Maker's up there winking in the rising of the sun,

Saying, "Morning to you, child! Look at all we've just begun!"

So leave the heavy worries at the bottom of the stairs,

We've got a spectacular today, a gift beyond compare.

Yeah, I'm dancing in the daylight, I've got nothing left to fear,

Spectacular is waiting... Spectacular is here!

Outro

Spectacular is waiting... Oh, the morning's bright and clear!

Spectacular is waiting... Spectacular is here!

Acknowledgments / About the Author

Henry is a father, caregiver, engineer, patent attorney, real estate broker, entrepreneur, and lifelong learner.

Over a 40-year career beginning in the early 1980s, Henry focused on advancing telecommunications technology in Dallas, Texas. His work evolved from engineering positions to operational leadership as he developed innovations in high-speed mobility and wireless connectivity.

Outside of work, Henry is a devoted husband and father, as you'll read in this book. He's also an award-winning business leader and entrepreneur whose mentorship has enabled colleagues worldwide to achieve significant professional growth. People recognize him for driving innovation, tackling complex challenges, and raising industry standards. Many who worked with him recall the industry 'firsts' he helped make possible.

Henry thanks lifelong friends David Walsh, Charles A. Sowders II, Richard Pratt, and mentor Joe McBride, whose trust was pivotal. Henry credits Joe's belief for many good things in his career.

Henry studied Electrical Engineering at Texas A&M University, then earned a law degree and completed extra certificates in management and finance. Top international companies trusted him to lead engineering and operations teams worldwide. His impact on the mobile broadband industry is still felt today.

Another special group has supported Henry for over 30 years, beginning with a connection in Jamaica in the mid-1990s that has since become a lifelong friendship. Soon after his wedding, Henry felt called to serve as a short-term missionary across the U.S., South America, and the Caribbean. On these trips, he met two men sharing the gospel through a film based on Luke, sponsored by the Bass family from Fort Worth. Inspired, Henry joined the effort, meeting people like Dave Hannah, Dave McDowell, and Steve Douglas, among others, who spread grace worldwide. Henry has since contributed his time, resources, and skills to these missions.

Henry started his entrepreneurial journey in 1992 with partners Darrel, David, Tom H., and Tom W. Later, Fred H. joined the group. Since then, Henry has pursued new business ventures with determination. Over time, his partnership with

David Kaltenbach grew into a relationship built on trust and shared values. After his divorce, Fred Harkins became a loyal friend, especially helping Henry and Taylor.

Henry is deeply grateful to the doctors, therapists, and educators who have supported our family. On behalf of Taylor and the family, he thanks you for your loyalty, kindness, and dedication.

Most importantly, Taylor's doctors are extraordinary. Dr. Patricia Evans and Dr. Frank E. Ford, your steady care, guidance, and encouragement have helped keep Taylor healthy, strong, safe, and comforted. I am deeply grateful for your commitment to her and to families like ours.

Each group of men has been vital to Henry's growth as a person, husband, father, and business leader. Henry keeps his circle small and remains loyal, a lasting friend who stands the test of time. Once you know him, it's often for life.

The End

Visit the author's web site

www.ingramcontent.com/pod-product-compliance
Lightning Source LLC
LaVergne TN
LVHW010840120826
845149LV00017B/3411
9798995720744